The Sheldon Short Guide to
Heart Attacks

Mark Greener spent a decade in biomedical research before joining *MIMS Magazine* for GPs in 1989. Since then, he has written on health and biology for magazines worldwide for patients, healthcare professionals and scientists. He is a member of the Royal Society of Biology and is the author of 21 other books, including *The Heart Attack Survival Guide* (2012) and *The Holistic Health Handbook* (2013), both published by Sheldon Press. Mark lives with his wife, three children and two cats in a Cambridgeshire village.

GW00708142

Sheldon Short Guides

A list of titles in the Overcoming Common Problems series is also available from Sheldon Press, 36 Causton Street, London SW1P 4ST and on our website at www.sheldonpress.co.uk

THE SHELDON SHORT GUIDE TO
HEART ATTACKS

Mark Greener

sheldon PRESS

First published in Great Britain in 2016

Sheldon Press
36 Causton Street
London SW1P 4ST
www.sheldonpress.co.uk

The author and publisher have made every effort to
ensure that the external website and email addresses
included in this book are correct and up to date at the
time of going to press. The author and publisher are
not responsible for the content, quality or continuing
accessibility of the sites.

British Library Cataloguing-in-Publication Data
A catalogue record for this book is available from the
British Library

ISBN 978–1–84709–384–4
eBook ISBN 978–1–84709–385–1

Typeset by Fakenham Prepress Solutions, Fakenham,
Norfolk NR21 8NN
First printed in Great Britain by Ashford Colour Press
Subsequently digitally reprinted in Great Britain

eBook by Fakenham Prepress Solutions, Fakenham,
Norfolk NR21 8NN

Produced on paper from sustainable forests

Contents

A note to the reader

This is not a medical book and is not intended to replace advice from your doctor. Consult your pharmacist or doctor if you believe you have any of the symptoms described, and if you think you might need medical help.

A note on references

I used numerous medical and scientific papers to write the book that this Sheldon Short is based on: *The Heart Attack Survival Guide*. Unfortunately, there isn't space to include references in this short summary. You can find these in *The Heart Attack Survival Guide,* which discusses the topics in more detail. I updated some facts and figures for this book.

Introduction

Every three minutes someone in the UK suffers a heart attack, according to the British Heart Foundation (BHF; <www.bhf.org.uk>). Indeed, cardiovascular (heart and circulatory) disease kills about 160,000 people a year. While improved treatments and greater awareness of risk factors helped reduce deaths from heart disease over recent decades, millions of people in the UK are at risk of suffering their first myocardial infarction (MI), the medical term for a heart attack. Once you survive one heart attack, you may well face another. But you can reduce your risk – even if you've developed angina, suffered an MI or are in your autumn years.

Almost anyone can suffer a heart attack. But some people are especially vulnerable. According to INTERHEART, a worldwide investigation into MI risk factors:

- People with diabetes who smoke and have hypertension (dangerously raised blood pressure) are 13 times more likely to suffer an MI than those without any of these three risk factors.
- Add a harmful profile of fat in your blood and obesity to these three risk factors and you're almost 69 times more likely to have a heart attack.
- Suffer psychosocial problems (such as severe stress at home or work, or depression) in addition to the five other risk factors and you are 334 times more likely to suffer a heart attack than those without any of these risk factors.

Following the advice in this book and that offered by your doctor, nurse or pharmacist can dramatically improve your heart's health, even if you've suffered a heart attack or unstable angina – which is a dangerous 'first cousin' to MI. An MI doesn't need to break your heart.

1

The heart of the matter

The average healthy heart is about the size of your fist, weighs around 0.3 kilograms (10 ounces) and pumps blood along 60,000 miles of vessels. Incredibly, if you laid your blood vessels end to end they'd go around the equator almost two and a half times. At rest, a healthy heart typically pumps 60 to 80 times a minute moving about 11,000 litres (2,500 gallons) of blood a day. Blood vessels form two 'circulatory systems' that begin and end at the heart (Figure 1):

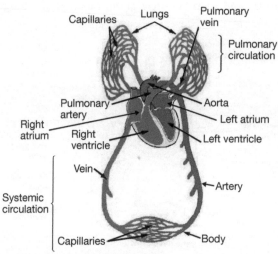

Figure 1 The circulatory system

- The pulmonary circulation connects your heart to your lungs.
- The systemic circulation connects your heart to all other parts of your body.

The heart's four chambers – two atria and two ventricles (Figure 2) – beat in sequence, pushing blood around the circulation:

- Systole refers to the contraction of the heart's chambers.
- Diastole is the relaxation between beats, when the chambers fill with blood.

So, doctors and nurses record systolic and diastolic blood pressure.

The atria collect blood from the circulation and, when they contract, push blood into the ventricles, helping the larger chambers work effectively. The right atrium and right ventricle pump blood to the lungs.

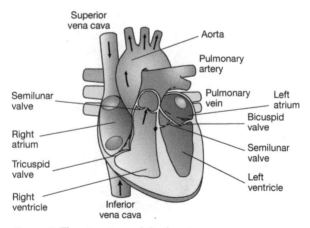

Figure 2 The structure of the heart

The left atrium and left ventricle pump blood to the rest of the body. So, the left ventricle is larger. Seven in every ten heart attacks occur in the left ventricle.

Controlling the flow

Heart valves ensure correct blood flow (Figure 2):

- Tricuspid valves control blood flow between the right atrium and right ventricle.
- Bicuspid (mitral) valves control blood flow between the left atrium and left ventricle.
- Semilunar valves prevent blood in the arteries from flowing back into the ventricles.

Early in diastole, the bicuspid and the tricuspid valves (together called the atrioventricular valves) open. Blood drains into the ventricles. After the ventricles are about three-quarters full, the atria contract. This forces the rest of the blood into the ventricles.

As the heart contracts, the bicuspid and tricuspid valves close to stop the pressure from forcing blood into the atria. As the pressure increases further, the semilunar valves (sometimes called the pulmonary valve and the aortic valve) open. Blood flows into two large blood vessels: the pulmonary artery and the aorta. The semilunar valves close at the beginning of diastole, which prevents blood from flowing back into the ventricles.

Controlling the beat

A pacemaker – the sinoatrial node – generates the heart's rhythm. Nerves and some chemical messages (e.g. hormones) 'fine tune' the rhythm to meet your body's needs. The sinoatrial node generates a pulse of

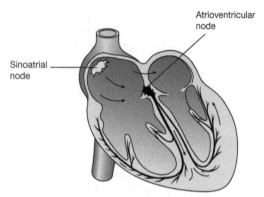

Atrioventricular node

Sinoatrial node

Figure 3 A wave of electrical activity keeps your heart's chambers beating in sequence

electricity that spreads through the muscle to ensure that the heart contracts in sequence (Figure 3). Doctors measure this wave using an electrocardiogram (ECG).

The circulatory system

Blood from the body, rich in carbon dioxide, enters the right atrium through two large veins: the superior vena cava and the inferior vena cava (Figure 2). The right atrium pumps blood into the right ventricle. When the heart contracts, blood flows from the right ventricle into the pulmonary artery, which splits into two to supply each lung. Carbon dioxide moves from the blood into the lungs and is expelled when we breathe out. Meanwhile, oxygen in the air we've breathed in attaches to an iron-rich protein (haemoglobin) in red blood cells (erythrocytes). Oxygen-rich blood travels to the left atrium.

Arteries, veins and capillaries

Arteries carry blood from the heart and branch into medium-sized and then small arteries (arterioles). These 'arterioles' divide into microscopic capillaries. These tiny vessels have thin walls that allow oxygen and nutrients to move from the blood into the tissue. Meanwhile, blood in the capillaries absorbs carbon dioxide and other waste products. (In the lung, oxygen moves into the capillaries, while carbon dioxide moves out.) Capillaries merge, forming venules and, in turn, veins that return blood to the heart. Most arteries carry oxygen-rich blood. Most veins carry oxygen-depleted blood. However, pulmonary arteries carry oxygen-poor blood from your heart to your lungs. Pulmonary veins return oxygen-rich blood.

The left ventricle pumps blood into the ascending aorta (Figure 2). From here, the blood takes one of four routes:

- Coronary arteries supply the heart (cardiac) muscle with oxygen and nutrients. Angina (page 8) occurs when the heart's demand for oxygen outstrips the supply. Most heart attacks occur when a blockage in the coronary circulation stops blood flow.
- Carotid arteries carry blood along the neck to the brain's cerebral circulation.
- The thoracic aorta supplies the chest, the head, the arms and hands.
- The abdominal aorta supplies organs between the chest and pelvis, as well as the legs and feet.

Controlling heart rate

Pacemakers (Figure 3) mean that your heart beats independently of nervous control. Nerves and hormones 'fine tune' the rate and force of the heartbeat. Your brain and spinal cord make up your central nervous system (CNS). Biologists divide nerves outside the CNS into:

- The 'somatic' or 'voluntary' nervous system, which allows us to choose actions.
- The 'autonomic' or 'involuntary' nervous system, which keeps functions like breathing and heartbeat going without conscious control, such as while we're asleep.

Changes in breathing can alter heart rate by 12 to 15 beats per minute. So, taking deep breaths can help you feel calmer. As more oxygen reaches your blood your heart doesn't need to work as hard. Nerves tell your brain that the heart's rate and force has declined. It's hard to feel mentally stressed when your body relaxes.

More than plumbing

Blood vessels have three layers:

- tunica intima, the smooth inner lining;
- tunica media, the middle layer, which controls the vessel's diameter and maintains its flexibility; and
- tunica adventitia (or tunica externa), which maintains the vessel's shape and anchors the vessel to nearby organs.

Each heartbeat generates sufficient force to send blood spurting feet into the air. The tunica media in arteries is much thicker than in veins to withstand the extra force. Arteries expand to accommodate the surge of blood. Your pulse is the pressure wave generated as blood travels along the arteries.

Blood pressure gradually weakens as arteries divide into arterioles and capillaries. By the time capillaries form veins, there's little pressure left to push blood to the heart. So, the tunica intima folds over, forming valves that prevent blood from flowing towards your ankles. Weak or damaged valves allow blood to flow backwards, causing varicose (enlarged, swollen) veins.

2

When a heart attack strikes

Smears of fat inside blood vessels start from child-hood – perhaps even while we are in the womb. This accumulation – atherosclerosis – causes most heart attacks. 'Sclerosis' means hardening, and 'athere' gruel or porridge. I'll never forget the film at a medical conference where a cardiac surgeon ran his finger along the outside of an artery with severe atherosclerosis. Fat ran out as if he was squeezing toothpaste from a tube.

Over time, these 'smears' of fat develop into plaques (see page 9), which often take 10 to 15 years to mature fully. As a plaque enlarges, the lumen (the 'bore' down the middle) narrows (Figure 4). This reduces the blood flow, which can cause:

- *Angina* A plaque in the coronary circulation reduces blood flow to the heart. Exercise and stress increase the heart's demand for oxygen. So, a plaque can trigger chest pain during exercise or when you're emotionally stressed (stable angina). The pain forces you to rest or calm down, which rebalances supply and demand. Doctors call plaques in the coronary circulation coronary artery disease, ischaemic heart disease or coronary heart disease (CHD).
- *Peripheral artery disease* Plaques can form in arteries supplying your limbs. The reduced blood supply

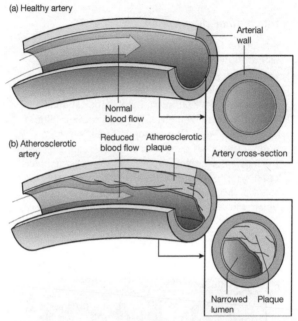

(a) Healthy artery

Arterial wall

Normal blood flow

Artery cross-section

(b) Atherosclerotic artery

Reduced blood flow

Atherosclerotic plaque

Narrowed lumen   Plaque

Figure 4 Atherosclerotic plaques can reduce the lumen of a blood vessel

to your legs – the most common site of peripheral atherosclerosis – can cause intermittent claudication (see box overleaf).

- *Stroke* Plaques can develop inside arteries supplying the brain, which can lead to strokes.

Plaque development

Fat collects around damage to the tunica intima (Figure 5 overleaf) following, for example:

- turbulent blood flow, such as around branches in vessels;

Intermittent claudication

Intermittent claudication is aching or cramping pain, with tightness or fatigue in leg muscles or buttocks. Sometimes the pain arises only during strenuous activity. People with more severe peripheral arterial disease may develop intermittent claudication after walking only a few metres. The pain subsides after a few minutes' rest. One person in three with coronary artery disease has peripheral arterial disease affecting the legs. Intermittent claudication can emerge before chest symptoms and may warn that you're likely to suffer an MI. Tell your doctor if you have leg pain when you walk or climb stairs.

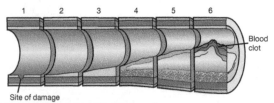

Blood clot

Site of damage

1 Damage to the inner lining of the blood vessel
2 Fatty streak forms at site of damage
3 Numbers of white blood cells increase, area is inflamed and small pools of fat appear
4 Large core of fat develops, and amounts of muscle and collagen increase
5 Fibrous cap covers a fat-rich core, while calcium deposits harden the plaque
6 Plaque ruptures, triggering a blood clot

Figure 5 Development of an atherosclerotic plaque

- high levels of fat in the blood (dyslipidaemia);
- raised sugar levels in the blood (diabetes);
- hypertension;
- changes linked to age;
- nicotine and other toxins from smoking; and
- inflammation that spreads from diseases in other parts of the body.

The damage allows fats and certain white blood cells to enter the vessel wall. Some white blood cells engorge with fat, forming foam cells. Meanwhile, chemicals released by white blood cells promote inflammation around the damage and increase the amount of muscle and collagen in the vessel wall. (Collagen enhances strength and flexibility.) The chemicals attract even more white blood cells to the damaged area.

These changes 'patch' the damage. But fat continues to pour from the blood into the plaque. So, muscle cells form a fibrous cap covering a core of foam cells, lipid and debris from dead cells. Capillaries grow into the developing plaque. So, blood leaks into, and further swells, the plaque. Calcium deposits gradually harden the plaque.

A silent killer

At first, arteries enlarge to accommodate the plaque. But after the plaque occupies more than 40 per cent of the vessel wall, it begins to narrow the lumen and cuts blood flow. Once a plaque blocks 50–70 per cent of the lumen, blood flow falls sufficiently to produce angina.

Sometimes, however, even marked declines in blood flow don't cause symptoms. Between 1 in 50 and 1 in 25 of us show this 'silent ischaemia', a figure that can exceed four in five of heart attack survivors.

Even MIs can be 'silent': the person may show changes in ECG (page 32), blood tests (page 32) and so on that are characteristic of a heart attack without symptoms. In other people, the symptoms are so mild that they're dismissed as, for instance, indigestion. Patients may discover they've suffered a heart attack after undergoing a test for another problem or during a 'routine' check-up. Indeed, a study from the USA found that almost one in 12 middle-aged and elderly people showed scars on their heart, which are almost always caused by MIs. But doctors have detected only one in five of the events causing the scar.

Plaque rupture

So-called stable plaques may not change for years. In other cases, inflammation weakens the plaque, which becomes unstable. Once the plaque has weakened sufficiently, factors such as exercise, increased blood pressure or changes in the blood vessel's diameter can rupture the plaque. This triggers a clot that can block the blood vessel. Plaque rupture causes seven in every ten heart attacks and cases of unstable angina, a related disease. Most other heart attacks follow the cap's slow erosion. Again, the contents leak into the blood, triggering a clot.

Plaques can also cause:

- *Stable angina* The heart's demand for oxygen outstrips supply – such as during exercise or intense emotion. However, no clot blocks the vessel, resting restores the balance and the heart muscle isn't damaged.
- *Unstable angina* A clot partially blocks the vessel. So, resting doesn't restore the balance. However,

the heart isn't damaged. Unstable angina produces similar symptoms to stable angina, but typically emerges at rest, and is more severe and prolonged – lasting longer than 20 minutes – than stable angina.

Don't ignore any warning signs. About 30 per cent of people have a heart attack within three months of suffering unstable angina:

- Go to A&E if you suffer symptoms that could be unstable angina.
- Tell your doctor immediately (or go to A&E) if your pattern of angina changes, such as from symptoms after exercise to symptoms while watching the television.

Limiting the damage

In around two-thirds of heart attacks and unstable angina attacks, the body removes the clot within 24 hours and repairs the damage, helping the heart muscle recover. But a blockage lasting for more than 20 minutes starts irreversibly damaging the heart. If the blockage lasts between six and eight hours, most of the muscle supplied by the vessel has died.

A few days after the MI, scar tissue starts replacing damaged muscle. The scar tissue does not contract as well as healthy muscle, which in some people leads to breathlessness, tiredness and swollen ankles – the hallmarks of heart failure (page 44) – and causes tell-tale changes on ECGs. In addition, many plaques remain unstable. Furthermore, few heart attack survivors have a single plaque. As people who have had a heart attack are at high risk of suffering another MI, you need to tackle the underlying disease.

Cardiac arrest

During a cardiac arrest, the heart stops pumping blood. The person loses consciousness almost immediately and won't breathe normally. Several events can trigger cardiac arrest, including heart attacks, electrocution, choking, losing large amounts of blood, being very hot or cold, and ventricular fibrillation.

Heart attacks can cause ventricular fibrillation, the most common cause of cardiac arrest. During ventricular fibrillation, the heart's electrical activity becomes chaotic. The ventricles stop pumping and 'quiver' (fibrillate). Defibrillators deliver an electric shock through the chest wall, which sometimes restores normal beats. If you think someone is in cardiac arrest, call 999 immediately, give cardiopulmonary resuscitation and, if you are trained, use a defibrillator; these are increasingly common in offices, public venues and shopping malls.

Heart attack triggers

A study published in *The Lancet* in 2011 analysed 36 studies assessing the risk of suffering a heart attack between two hours and a day after encountering a variety of triggers. Cocaine increased heart attack risk 24 times. Other triggers included a heavy meal (a sevenfold increase), exercise (a fourfold increase) and sex (a threefold increase). Speak to your doctor or rehabilitation team about avoiding situations that could precipitate a heart attack.

Anaemia and heart attacks

Depending on the people studied and the definitions, up to two in every five MI patients have anaemia. In other words, they have too little haemoglobin, the iron-containing protein in red blood cells that carries oxygen. Causes include:

- producing too few or destroying too many red blood cells;
- deficiencies in vitamin B_{12}, iron or folic acid;
- long-lasting inflammation;
- certain cancers.

Anaemic people may feel fatigued and weak, suffer headache and palpitations, feel breathless and find that exercise becomes more difficult. Low haemoglobin levels further undermine oxygen supply, which exacerbates any heart damage and can cause severe chest pain. So, the heart works harder and the left ventricle thickens (left ventricular hypertrophy).

Anaemia increases the risk of death among people with heart failure (page 44) and after a heart attack. So, ask your doctor to measure your haemoglobin level. You could also consider taking a multivitamin and eating foods rich in vitamin B_{12}, iron or folic acid. Ask your GP or a dietician or look at the British Dietetic Association website (<www.bda.uk.com>).

3

Risk factors for heart attacks

You can't do much about some of the 200–300 heart attack risk factors – such as your age and sex. But nine easily measured and potentially modifiable risk factors account for about nine in every ten first heart attacks.

These nine factors emerged from the landmark INTERHEART study, published in *The Lancet* in 2004, which compared 15,152 people from 52 countries who'd suffered their first heart attack with 14,820 people who'd never experienced an MI. INTERHEART found that:

- Smoking almost trebled the chances of suffering an MI. Smoking one to five cigarettes a day increased the risk by 38 per cent compared to lifelong non-smokers. The risk roughly doubled in those smoking six to ten cigarettes a day, increased almost fourfold between 16 and 20 a day, and rose to just over nine-fold in people smoking at least 41 cigarettes a day.
- Diabetes and hypertension each roughly doubled the risk of the first heart attack.
- High levels of harmful fats in the blood increased MI risk up to threefold (Table 1).
- Abdominal obesity ('a bulging waistline') increased the risk up to about 60 per cent.
- Psychosocial factors (such as stress and depression) roughly trebled the risk.

On the other hand, eating fruits and vegetables daily (30 per cent reduction), regular exercise (14 per cent reduction) and regular alcohol consumption (9 per cent reduction) protected against the first heart attack.

So, eliminating smoking would prevent just over a third of first MIs. Eliminating abnormal fat levels would almost halve the number of first heart attacks. Hypertension and abdominal obesity accounted for almost a fifth of MIs, and diabetes for one in ten.

Many risk factors 'cluster'. Fat is packed with calories. So, if you eat a high-fat diet, for example, you're more likely to be overweight. And the risk of an MI rises dramatically the more risk factors you have:

- People with diabetes who smoke and have hypertension are 13 times more likely to suffer a heart attack than those without any of the nine risk factors.

Table 1 Factors linked to the risk of suffering the first heart attack in the INTERHEART study

Risk factors	Increase in risk of MI
Hypertension alone	2 times
Diabetes alone	2 times
Smoking alone	3 times
Abnormal lipid profile (ApoB/A1 ratio)	3 times
Hypertension, diabetes, smoking	13 times
Hypertension, diabetes, smoking, adverse lipids	42 times
Hypertension, diabetes, smoking, adverse lipids, obesity	69 times
Hypertension, diabetes, smoking, adverse lipids, psychosocial factors	183 times
Hypertension, diabetes, smoking, adverse lipids, psychosocial factors, obesity	334 times

Source: Adapted from Yusuf S, et al. Lancet 2004;364: 937–52.

- Those with five risk factors (harmful fat levels, obesity, smoking, diabetes and hypertension) are almost 69 times more likely to have a heart attack.
- If you have psychosocial risk factors in addition to these other five risk factors you are about 334 times more likely to suffer a heart attack than those without any of the nine risk factors.

Stress and heart attacks

INTERHEART assessed the link between stress – feeling irritable, anxious or having difficulty sleeping because of problems – and MIs. The researchers separated, as far as possible:

- stress at work
- stress at home
- stress caused by financial problems
- major stressful life events (such as divorce, business failure, unemployment or death of a spouse).

After allowing for other risk factors, such as age, sex and smoking:

- People who experienced several periods of work-related stress were 38 per cent more likely to suffer a heart attack.
- Experiencing several periods of stress at home increased the risk by 52 per cent.
- Heart attack risk roughly doubled in those who endured permanent stress at work or home.
- Severe financial stress increased the likelihood of a first MI by 33 per cent.
- Stressful life events increased first MI risk by 48 per cent.
- Feeling depressed for at least two weeks in the year before the study increased MI risk by 55 per cent.

Psychologists describe the extent to which you feel you control your life as your 'locus of control'.

- If you have a strong external locus of control, you see yourself as having little influence over your life. You feel that events control you, you don't control events.
- A strong internal locus of control means you tend to see yourself as in charge of your life. People with a strong internal locus are, generally, less stressed than those with an external locus of control.

INTERHEART found that a high internal locus of control reduced MI risk by 32 per cent and that stress causes up to a third of heart attacks. In other words, psychological factors are as important as hypertension and obesity as a cause of heart attacks.

Metabolic syndrome

'Metabolic syndrome' describes a particularly hazardous cluster of cardiovascular risk factors. Definitions vary, but if you have at least three of the following, a doctor may diagnose metabolic syndrome:

- a large waistline – abdominal obesity or 'an apple shape' – at least 94 cm (37 inches) in European men and at least 80 cm (32 inches) in European women (cut-offs differ for certain ethnic origins) (see Table 7 on page 63);
- abnormal lipids, such as low levels of high-density lipoprotein (HDL), or you're taking a medicine (ask your GP or pharmacist) to boost levels of this 'healthy' fat;
- high levels of triglycerides or you're taking medicines to cut levels of this harmful fat;
- hypertension or you're taking a medicine to reduce your blood pressure;

- diabetes or a high blood sugar level when you haven't eaten for several hours (an early sign of diabetes), or you are taking a drug for diabetes.

In INTERHEART, metabolic syndrome increases the risk of the first heart attack by 120 to 169 per cent. So, if you have one risk factor ask your GP or nurse to check for others.

Hypertension

Your blood pressure depends on the force generated by the heart, the amount of blood pumped around your circulation, and the size and flexibility of your arteries.

Doctors and nurses take two blood pressure readings. If your blood pressure is 120/80 mmHg:

- the top reading (120 mmHg) represents the peak systolic pressure as your heart contracts;
- the bottom reading (80 mmHg) is the lowest diastolic pressure when your heart relaxes between beats.

Blood pressure increases (e.g. during exercise) or decreases to meet your body's demands. In some people, however, blood pressure remains elevated when they're just sitting or lying down. Dangerously raised blood pressure is 'hypertension'.

If you suffer any of the symptoms in Table 2, you should see a doctor urgently. These could indicate an especially dangerous form called malignant hypertension. Usually, however, hypertension does not cause symptoms. So, unless your blood pressure is measured regularly, a stroke or MI may be the first sign you have hypertension.

Table 2 Symptoms that could indicate malignant hypertension

Headache – especially if severe
Confusion
Tinnitus, buzzing or noise in the ears
Fatigue
Irregular heartbeat
Nosebleed, without injury
Changes in vision

Hypertension can damage arteries, triggering the formation of fatty streaks, or rupture plaques. INTERHEART showed that hypertension roughly doubles MI risk and causes almost a fifth of heart attacks. Hypertension also contributes to almost three-quarters of strokes.

Doctors can identify an underlying cause in only 1 in 20 to 1 in 10 cases of dangerously raised blood pressure (secondary hypertension). Treating underlying causes – such as some kidney diseases, Cushing's syndrome (a rare hormonal disease), sleep apnoea and some drugs – often lowers blood pressure to safe levels. Most people will, however, need to take antihypertensives – drugs that lower blood pressure – and make lifestyle changes to control blood pressure and reduce MI risk.

A doctor or nurse should measure your blood pressure at least once a year. You can buy a blood pressure monitor to use at home, but make sure it's accurate and you have the right-sized cuff. Your GP or hospital, the BHF or the Blood Pressure Association (<www.blood pressureuk.org>) may be able to help.

Lethal and healthy cholesterol

Despite its bad press, we need cholesterol. It's an essential building block of the membranes that surround every cell, forms part of the insulation (myelin sheath) around many nerves that ensures that signals travel properly, and is the backbone of several hormones. But poor diet and a lack of exercise (which burns fat) mean that many of us have too much of a good thing.

To transport cholesterol, your body surrounds a core of fat with soluble coats called lipoproteins. For example:

- Low-density lipoprotein (LDL) carries cholesterol from the liver to the tissues. LDL accumulates in artery walls, contributing to atherosclerosis.
- HDL carries cholesterol away from the arteries and back to the liver for excretion. HDL removes cholesterol from plaques, slowing atherosclerosis.

In other words, high LDL levels increase heart attack risk. High levels of HDL protect against MIs. It's easy to remember: LDL is 'lethal'; HDL is 'healthy'. Your doctor will probably measure more than total cholesterol – such as the balance between HDL and LDL, triglycerides and very low density lipoprotein (VLDL) – to optimize treatment.

Triglycerides: the other fat

Your body converts carbohydrates (such as starch and sugar) into a sugar called glucose. Your body uses glucose as fuel. You turn leftover glucose into triglycerides, which you store in fat cells. If you don't burn the energy stores, you pile on the pounds. Several factors – including smoking, diabetes, obesity and metabolic syndrome – increase triglyceride levels.

Lipoproteins rich in triglycerides easily enter damaged artery walls. As they're larger than LDL, they're more likely to remain in the plaque, where, for example, they trigger inflammation and hinder the breakdown of blood clots. People with high triglyceride levels in their blood tend to have low levels of HDL, and vice versa.

Diabetes

The hormone insulin helps cells take up glucose, which they use for energy. If your pancreas does not produce enough insulin or the hormone does not work properly (insulin resistance), the glucose in your blood rises to dangerously high levels that poison cells. Over several years, the raised levels of sugar can cause debilitating, distressing and disabling complications, such as pain, ulcers, amputations, heart disease and blindness. The body tries to reduce blood glucose levels by flushing the excess out. So, people with diabetes urinate more and experience a range of other symptoms. See your doctor if you suffer any symptom in Table 3.

Table 3 Common symptoms of diabetes

More frequent urination than usual, especially at night
Increased thirst; drinking excessively
Extreme tiredness and fatigue
Unexplained weight loss
Genital itching or regular episodes of thrush
Cuts and wounds that heal slowly
Blurred vision

Doctors subdivide diabetes into two main types:

- *Type 1 diabetes* Our immune system targets harmful bacteria, viruses and parasites. To limit 'collateral' damage to healthy tissues, proteins called antibodies 'stick' to the invaders and trigger a targeted immune reaction. Occasionally, however, the immune system produces antibodies against healthy tissues (autoantibodies), a process called autoimmunity). Type 1 diabetes arises when antibodies destroy insulin-producing cells in the pancreas.
- *Type 2 diabetes (T2D)* This usually occurs in obese and overweight people aged more than 40 years.

Many of us have no idea that we've developed T2D. The first sign may be a heart attack or another serious complication, such as nerve pain, an ulcer or changes in vision. Indeed, by the time they're diagnosed, half of people with T2D have complications. In addition, T2D shortens life expectancy by up to ten years, largely because your risk of heart disease increases between two- and fourfold. Diabetes also cuts your chance of surviving a heart attack.

Sending your heart up in smoke

A cigarette smoker is nearly twice as likely to have a heart attack as a non-smoker. Younger people and women are especially vulnerable. Smokers under the age of 40 years are five times more likely to suffer a heart attack than their non-smoking peers, for example. Furthermore, in one study, smokers were 60 per cent more likely to die after they suffered a heart attack than non-smokers.

Smoking damages the heart in several ways:

- Nicotine makes the heart beat more rapidly and increases blood pressure.
- Tobacco smoke is rich in carbon monoxide, which reduces the blood's ability to carry oxygen. So, the heart needs to work harder.
- Smoking increases levels of cholesterol in the blood and undermines the balance between 'healthy' HDL and 'lethal' LDL.
- Smoking increases the risk of blood clots.

On the other hand, MI risk halves within a year of quitting. People who quit reduce their risk of dying from the disease by about 40 per cent.

Excess weight and obesity

Excess weight is a leading cause of heart disease: even gaining just 5 kg may increase CHD risk by 30 per cent. In addition, obesity and several other heart attack risk factors are intimately linked. For example:

- Hypertension is between five and six times more common in obese people (those with a body mass index – BMI – over 30 kg/m^2) compared to those of healthy BMI (18.5–24.9 kg/m^2).
- Excess weight causes around 90 per cent of cases of T2D.
- Obesity is a core component of the metabolic syndrome.
- Triglycerides store energy in fat cells.

But weight isn't a very good guide to your risk of developing MI or other diseases linked to excess weight. Weighing 90 kg (about 14 stone) is fine if you're 2 metres (about 6 foot 6 inches) tall, but you're seriously obese if you're 1.7 metres (about 5 foot 6 inches). So, BMI assesses whether you're overweight or obese based on your height and weight. You can use an on-line calculator (see <www.nhs.uk/Tools/Pages/Healthyweightcalculator.aspx>) or ask your doctor, pharmacist or nurse to calculate your BMI.

Try to keep your BMI between 18.5 and 24.9 kg/m^2. Below this and you're dangerously underweight. A BMI between 25.0 and 29.9 kg/m^2 suggests that you are overweight. You're probably obese if your BMI exceeds 30.0 kg/m^2. However, BMI may overestimate body fat in muscular people. On the other hand, BMI may underestimate body fat in older persons and others who have lost muscle. You doctor can check your body fat level.

Persistently raised heart rate

Persistently raised heart rate – even if not an arrhythmia – increases the risk of cardiovascular disease and death as much as smoking, raised cholesterol and hypertension. Deaths from any cause approximately double. On the other hand, regular exercise reduces heart rate.

Early heart attacks

Familial hypercholesterolaemia (FH) is an inherited disorder that causes high blood cholesterol from birth. So, a person with FH often suffers a heart attack relatively young. Yet 85 per cent of those affected don't know they have FH. Several less common genetic disorders also affect blood cholesterol levels.

Chronic kidney disease

In the UK, diabetes and hypertension are the leading causes of chronic kidney disease. People with diabetes excrete sugar in urine, which can damage their kidneys. Hypertension can damage blood vessels in the kidneys. So, diabetes and hypertension undermine the kidneys' ability to excrete waste and superfluous fluid. The extra fluid pushes blood pressure higher. Unless treated, the person may eventually need a kidney transplant or dialysis. So, cardiovascular disease increases the risk of kidney disease and kidney disease can increase the risk of cardiovascular disease.

Most of us are born with more kidney function than we need. So, mild chronic kidney disease doesn't usually cause symptoms. As kidney disease progresses you may develop several symptoms including:

- tiredness;
- swollen ankles, feet or hands;
- shortness of breath;
- itchy skin;
- nausea;
- problems having or keeping an erection.

See your doctor if you develop any of these symptoms.

If you have kidney disease you excrete protein in your urine (albuminuria or proteinuria). Using a dipstick to test for small increases in levels of albumin – the commonest blood protein – in the urine (microalbuminuria) can identify kidney disease long before you develop symptoms. Certain drugs slow the progression. So, check whether you've been tested recently.

Gout

Few diseases match the pain caused by gout. The Reverend Sydney Smith, a nineteenth-century wit, described his attacks as like 'walking on eyeballs'. Gout occurs when crystals of a chemical called sodium urate deposit in the joints. Gout attacks typically develop rapidly, often beginning at night in a single joint.

Numerous CHD risk factors increase the likelihood of developing gout, including:

- drinking alcohol;
- being overweight or obese;
- chronic kidney disease;
- heart failure;
- hypertension;
- raised levels of triglycerides or cholesterol.

4

Diagnosing heart attacks

Even experienced doctors can find MIs surprisingly difficult to diagnose. Not everyone develops the classic 'ischaemic' symptoms (e.g. pain or discomfort in the chest, abdomen, wrist or jaw). So, doctors use several techniques to determine whether you've suffered an MI. Early treatment offers your best chance of surviving an MI: if in doubt call 999.

The pain or discomfort caused by a heart attack usually begins in the centre or left side of the chest, then spreads to the arm, jaw, back or shoulder. The pain tends to be diffuse rather than sharp and confined to a small area. Heart attacks may trigger breathlessness, heavy sweating, nausea, vomiting or light-headedness. Moving the muscles around the site of the discomfort, taking a deep breath or changing position doesn't usually help.

- The discomfort caused by a heart attack can occur with or without exertion and does not usually go away with rest.
- In contrast, exertion or emotions tend to trigger stable angina, which subsides on rest.
- In general, the pain of a heart attack is more persistent than that of stable angina. But these aren't hard-and-fast rules.

Around two-thirds of people experience symptoms, including shortness of breath and fatigue, in the days to weeks before they suffer an MI. Stable angina may suddenly become more frequent or more severe, may last for longer or be provoked by less intense activity – so-called 'crescendo angina'. Remain alert for warning signs, such as a change in your pattern of angina, and see your GP as soon as possible.

When to call 999

If you suffer chest pain or other symptoms that you think could mean you're suffering a heart attack and your doctor has diagnosed angina, stop what you are doing, sit down and rest. Take your anti-angina spray or tablets. If the pain doesn't ease within five minutes, take your angina treatment again. Call 999 if the pain does not ease within five minutes of the second dose. Even if it does abate, see your GP.

If you haven't been diagnosed with angina (or you don't have your medicine) and suffer symptoms that could suggest a heart attack, sit down and rest. Take an aspirin if one is to hand, unless your doctor has told you not to, to help prevent blood clots. Call 999 if the pain doesn't go away in a couple of minutes. Even if the pain resolves, see your GP as soon as you can.

Atypical symptoms

Many people experience unusual (so-called 'atypical') symptoms during heart attacks. An MI may cause pain in the upper abdomen, for instance, which is easily confused with indigestion. MIs may cause pain in the arm, shoulder, wrist, jaw or back without chest discomfort. Atypical heart attacks are especially common in people aged 25–40 years and over 75 years of age, women and those with diabetes, chronic kidney disease, dementia, unstable angina or an NSTEMI (a type of MI). For instance, people with unstable angina or an NSTEMI may report:

- abdominal pain;
- bouts of indigestion;
- sharp stabbing chest pain, which may be worse when they breathe in;
- increasing breathlessness.

As doctors cannot rely on symptoms alone, they use tests including characteristic changes in certain enzymes and ECG changes to diagnose MIs. They may also use imaging techniques to locate the blocked coronary artery. Each test adds a piece to the jigsaw that leads the doctor to diagnose an MI or unstable angina (Table 4).

Table 4 Features of heart attack revealed by different tests

Test	Feature
Examination of heart tissue under the microscope	Death of heart cells
Blood tests	Indicate damage to the heart
Electrocardiography	Changes may indicate ischaemia or loss of normal heart tissue
Imaging	Reduced or lost blood supply to the heart
	Abnormal motion of the heart wall

Blood tests

During an MI, oxygen starvation gradually kills the area of heart muscle supplied by the blocked vessel. The damaged muscles release a cocktail of proteins into the blood, which aids diagnosis. For example, measuring levels of cardiac troponins allows doctors to assess damage to heart muscle. Troponins are specialized proteins that help muscles contract. Levels of cardiac troponins offer a very sensitive marker of damage to heart muscle. For instance, doctors use cardiac troponins to distinguish unstable angina (when levels don't rise) from a heart attack.

Electrocardiogram (ECG)

ECGs measure the electrical wave that ensures normal heartbeats. So ECGs can:

- record heart rate;
- help diagnose MIs;
- detect problems with heart rhythm, such as arrhythmia;
- distinguish two important subtypes of MI;
- indicate the cause of, or changes produced by, heart failure (page 44).

Depending on the shape of the ECG, a doctor may diagnose one of two types of heart attack:

- ST-segment elevation MI (STEMI)
- non-ST-segment elevation MI (NSTEMI).

These two types of heart attack have different outlooks. For instance, death while in hospital may be more common following STEMI than with unstable angina and NSTEMI. Death rates were similar after six months. But after four years, people with unstable angina or NSTEMI were twice as likely to have died as those with STEMI. Unstable angina and NSTEMI tend to occur in people with more extensive disease in their coronary arteries, older people and those with other ailments, especially kidney disease and diabetes. So, the poorer long-term prospects are perhaps not surprising.

Usually, you'll have your ECG taken while lying down. But sometimes, your doctor may monitor your heart continuously as you get on with life over 24 hours (ambulatory ECG or Holter monitoring). If symptoms are less frequent, the doctor may use a 'cardiac event recorder' to record the heart's activity for longer or when symptoms occur.

Your doctor might use an ECG to see how well your heart works during activity, such as walking on a treadmill or pedalling a stationary bike. You'll gradually increase the exercise for, usually, up to 15 minutes. Tell the doctor, nurse or technician if you develop chest pain or discomfort, experience other symptoms or become very tired or breathless.

Imaging and angiography

Your doctor may suggest cardiac imaging to examine your heart, reveal blockages in your coronary circulation and evaluate your heart valves.

Cardiac imaging can help detect a heart attack or ischaemia, identify other conditions that cause chest pain, predict your prognosis and detect some complications. For instance, coronary arteries don't show up on X-rays. So, during 'angiography', the radiographer injects 'contrast medium' into your coronary arteries, which absorbs X-rays and reveals small blood vessels. The X-ray image (angiogram) can show the site and severity of any narrowing.

5

Treating heart attacks

MIs strike when the blood supply to part of the heart fails. So, treatment aims to restore blood flow, keep the vessels open and improve the supply of nutrients and oxygen to the damaged area (reperfusion). The sooner reperfusion begins, the better your chances.

Initially, paramedics and doctors will alleviate pain. In the ambulance, you may inhale oxygen or a mixture of nitrous oxide and oxygen (Entonox), and be offered other painkillers and, if you've not taken one already, an aspirin.

In A&E, a doctor or cardiac nurse specialist will assess your symptoms, record your history, measure your blood pressure and heart rate, perform an ECG, take a blood sample and use treatments to relieve symptoms and reduce the damage, such as:

- aspirin (if you've not received it previously);
- oxygen – increasing the amount of oxygen you breathe in means that your heart doesn't have to work as hard;
- morphine, the most effective painkiller;
- a nitrate injection, which opens coronary arteries and increases blood flow (a 'vasodilator'), so relieving chest pain and reducing heart damage;
- thrombolysis or coronary angioplasty with stents.

Aspirin

Aspirin targets small blood cells called platelets. When you start bleeding, platelets gather at the wound and stick together, forming a clot. The rupture of a plaque triggers platelets to clump inside the vessel. Aspirin reduces platelet aggregation and so cuts the risk of death from an MI. But never take aspirin – for a headache, for example – if you take other anticoagulants (see page 40) unless your doctor suggests the combination. You could risk excessive bleeding and even a stroke.

Once you leave hospital, you'll probably take aspirin every day to reduce your chance of suffering another MI. You will probably also take aspirin to help prevent your first heart attack if you are at high risk. You'll probably take another anti-platelet drug if you can't use aspirin.

Diuretics and ACE inhibitors

Your kidneys help control the amount of fluid in your urine and, in turn, your blood pressure. Your kidneys filter water, salts and some waste products from your blood. Diuretics ('water tablets') increase urine production. So, blood volume and pressure falls. In turn, your heart doesn't have to work as hard.

A chemical called aldosterone tells your kidneys to excrete less water, driving blood pressure up. To understand how ACE inhibitors work, we need to follow this pathway backwards.

A protein called angiotensin II triggers aldosterone release and narrows blood vessels, which increases blood pressure. In turn, an enzyme called ACE (angiotensin converting enzyme) converts a relatively inactive protein called angiotensin I into angiotensin

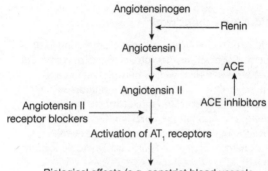

Figure 6 How ACE inhibitors work

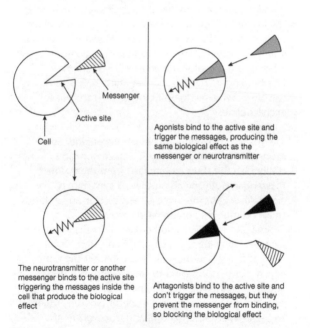

Figure 7 Drugs and receptors

How some drugs work

Numerous chemicals pass messages around your body. For example, neurotransmitters pass messages between nerves as well as between nerves and muscles. One neurotransmitter – noradrenaline – increases the force and rate at which the heart contracts. Another neurotransmitter – acetylcholine – has the opposite effect. The balance between the two helps match your heart's activity to your body's needs.

Many messengers bind to specific 'receptors'. Imagine a heart muscle cell as a car. The receptor is the ignition lock. The messenger – such as noradrenaline or acetylcholine – is the key. When the key fits into a lock, the engine starts (Figure 7). When the messenger binds to the receptor, part of the cell's internal machine starts. For example, angiotensin II binds to a receptor known as AT1 (Figure 6). This binding is specific: *your* key starts only *your* car. Noradrenaline doesn't bind to the receptor for acetylcholine.

Now imagine you have a skeleton key, which fits the ignition lock and switches on the engine. Some drugs act like a skeleton key. The receptor can't distinguish the drug (an agonist) from the normal messenger. Both switch on the cell's machinery. For example, adrenaline, which treats cardiac arrest, binds to and stimulates noradrenaline receptors.

Imagine you have another key. It fits the ignition lock but won't turn. So, the car won't start. But while this key is in the lock, you can't get the right key in. Some drugs bind to the receptor but don't activate the internal machinery. These are antagonists or 'blockers'. Angiotensin II receptor blockers, used to treat hypertension and heart failure, prevent angiotensin II from binding to AT1 receptors.

II (Figure 6). So, drugs that inhibit ACE reduce levels of angiotensin II and blood pressure declines.

Beta-blockers

Adrenaline and noradrenaline bind to beta-receptors, and so increase heart rate, strengthen the heart's contraction, narrow some blood vessels and stimulate renin release. In turn, renin converts a relatively inactive precursor into angiotensin I (Figure 6). Beta-blockers (beta-adrenergic receptor blockers) prevent adrenaline and noradrenaline from binding to this receptor. Overall, taken after a heart attack beta-blockers reduce total mortality, non-fatal MIs and sudden death by approximately 20 to 30 per cent. Beta-blockers are especially effective in people at high risk of another MI.

Thrombolytic drugs: the clot busters

A thrombolytic drug breaks down the blood clot (thrombus) blocking a blood vessel. This restores blood flow, limits further damage and encourages healing. So, doctors inject streptokinase or another thrombolytic as soon as they're sure you've suffered a heart attack.

The sooner blood flow is restored, the better your chances of surviving and the less damage your heart endures. Thrombolysis should normally begin within 12 hours of the start of symptoms of a heart attack. Ambulance paramedics may inject thrombolytic drugs.

Uncontrolled bleeding is the most important side effect: around one person in 100 receiving a thrombolytic suffers a stroke. Thrombolysis can cause poorly controlled bleeding at injection sites, in the gut or elsewhere, and dangerously low blood pressure. So, people with bleeding disorders (e.g. haemophilia) or who have recently haemorrhaged, been seriously injured, undergone surgery or suffered a recent stroke might not be suitable for thrombolysis.

Within two or three days, you'll produce antibodies, which may reduce the efficacy of subsequent streptokinase treatment and increase the risk of severe allergic reactions. If you've had streptokinase before, you (or your carer) should tell the ambulance or A&E team. Always carry your streptokinase card.

Heparin

Heparin keeps a blood clot from expanding or travelling to another part of your body. The original version – 'unfractionated heparin' – is often highly effective. But the response can fluctuate. So, people taking heparin need regular monitoring and often frequent dose changes. Used long term, unfractionated heparin can cause thrombocytopenia (abnormally low platelet numbers), uncontrolled bleeding and osteoporosis (brittle bone disease). The more recent low molecular weight heparins are more predictable, require less intensive monitoring and may be less likely to cause thrombocytopenia, bleeding and osteoporosis.

Glycoprotein IIb/IIIa inhibitors

Glycoprotein IIb/IIIa (GP IIb/IIIa) inhibitors prevent platelets from forming clots in certain people, such as:

- some of those who need angiography or percutaneous coronary intervention (PCI);
- people with unstable angina or NSTEMI, who are at high risk of a subsequent MI or death.

Calcium channel blockers

In addition to building strong bones and teeth, calcium ensures nerves and muscles work properly. For example, calcium allows the heart muscles and the rings of muscle that control the diameter of blood vessels (which maintain blood pressure) to contract. Calcium moves through proteins that form 'tunnels' through the membrane that surrounds each cell.

Calcium channel blockers (calcium antagonists) inhibit calcium's movement through these tunnels. The decline in calcium inside muscle cells dilates blood vessels and lowers blood pressure. Some calcium channel blockers reduce the force and rate of the heart's contraction.

Percutaneous coronary intervention (PCI)

During PCI, surgeons thread a thin catheter tipped with a balloon and guided by X-ray from an artery in the groin or arm to the blockage in the coronary artery. (The technique is also called percutaneous translu- minal coronary angioplasty, coronary artery balloon dilatation or balloon angioplasty.) Once the cath- eter is in place, the surgeon inflates the balloon, which compresses the plaque, widens the artery and improves blood flow. So, angioplasty can treat CHD and angina before an MI or if you develop angina after coronary artery bypass grafts (CABG; page 42). You'll need an angiogram before or at the same time as the angioplasty.

You'll probably be discharged from hospital after two or three days. Check the insertion site when you get home. You'll have some bruising. See your doctor if you get any redness or swelling or if the bruising worsens, and discuss with your doctor or nurse what you can do (e.g. work and exercise), and when, after angioplasty.

Occasionally, angioplasty may trigger an MI or stroke or completely block the coronary artery. So, around 1 in every 1,000 people undergoing angioplasty needs a coronary artery bypass graft (CABG). The area could become blocked again, which might mean another operation. So discuss the benefits and risks with a cardiologist.

Stents

A surgeon may slip a 'collapsed' stent – a wire frame – over the balloon catheter and move the tube next to the blockage. When the balloon inflates, the stent expands and remains in place, which improves blood flow and often relieves symptoms such as chest pain. Within a few weeks, the artery's inside lining covers the metal. So, blood flows easily over the stent without clotting. However, scar tissue forms underneath the healthy lining. In around a quarter of cases, thick scar tissue can obstruct blood flow (re-stenosis). Some stents release drugs that reduce re-stenosis. The concentration of these drugs is high around the stent but very little reaches the rest of the body. You'll probably also take aspirin and an antiplatelet drug to reduce the risk of clotting.

Coronary artery bypass graft (CABG)

CABG tends to be used when atherosclerosis causes severe narrowing or blockage of large coronary arteries. A double bypass refers to two grafts, a triple bypass to three grafts, quadruple to four and so on. Obviously, a quintuple bypass is much more serious than receiving a single graft.

The surgeon uses a section of healthy blood vessel from the leg, the chest or the arm to bypass the blocked coronary artery. You will need general anaesthesia, will probably spend several days in hospital and may take several months to recover fully.

Defibrillation

A heart attack can cause a marked disturbance in the heart's rhythm (arrhythmia). During ventricular fibrillation (page 14), the ventricles stop pumping and quiver uncontrollably ('fibrillate'), causing a cardiac arrest. An electric shock, using a defibrillator, often restores the normal heartbeat if administered quickly.

Automatic defibrillators, which diagnose the problem and deliver the appropriate pulse of electricity, are available increasingly in planes, at workplaces, in homes and in other locations. If an automated defibrillator isn't available, call 999 immediately and start cardiopulmonary resuscitation until the ambulance arrives. (Emergency ambulances carry defibrillators.) Paramedics may inject a person in cardiac arrest with adrenaline.

Unless defibrillation or cardiopulmonary resuscitation starts within three to four minutes the person may suffer permanent brain damage. If you're the partner or carer of someone with heart disease, learn cardiopulmonary resuscitation. Contact St John Ambulance (<www.sja.org.uk>) or the British Red Cross (<www.redcross.org.uk>).

6

After a heart attack

A fifth of survivors suffer another MI in the seven years after their first heart attack. So, treatment doesn't end when you're discharged from hospital. Taking your medicines as prescribed by your doctor and making lifestyle changes will dramatically reduce the risk of another heart attack. Modern medicines, although highly effective, do not replace a healthy lifestyle.

Heart failure

Heart failure arises when the heart 'fails' to pump enough blood to meet your body's demands. Doctors divide heart failure into two types. Eventually, most people with heart failure develop both.

- In left heart failure (left ventricular systolic dysfunction), the left ventricle cannot pump enough of the blood that it receives from the lungs. Blood backs up in the lungs (pulmonary oedema), causing breathlessness. This is potentially fatal.
- In right heart failure, the right ventricle cannot pump enough of the blood received from the body. So, blood backs up in the legs, ankles, torso and so on, causing peripheral oedema (congestion – congestive heart failure). This can cause puffiness of the hands, feet or face, discomfort and skin ulcers.

Heart failure can arise from:

- atherosclerosis in coronary arteries;
- scars on the heart left by MIs, which can prevent the heart from beating properly;
- excessive alcohol consumption;
- hypertension;
- congenital heart defects;
- infection of the heart valves (endocarditis) or heart muscle (myocarditis);
- left ventricular hypertrophy (LVH).

LVH describes the enlargement (hypertrophy) of the left ventricle caused when a disease or your lifestyle makes your heart work excessively hard for a long time. The ventricle thickens, becomes less elastic and eventually fails to pump with as much force as a healthy heart. LVH can follow, for example:

- hypertension, which is the most common cause of LVH: the left ventricle works harder to counter raised blood pressure;
- narrowing (stenosis) of the aortic valve;
- intense, prolonged endurance and strength training;
- obesity.

At first, you may not suffer symptoms. But as LVH progresses, you may experience shortness of breath, chest pain, palpitations, dizziness, fainting and rapid exhaustion with physical activity. The enlarged muscle may also compress coronary arteries, restricting the heart's blood supply and causing heart failure, arrhythmias, angina, cardiac arrest and MIs. There's not space here to discuss treatment for heart failure. So, contact your doctor, nurse or the BHF.

Arrhythmias

Arrhythmias are changes in the heart's rate or rhythm. The heart may beat too quickly (tachycardia), too slowly (bradycardia) or irregularly. For example, ventricular arrhythmias may cause cardiac arrest (page 13) and about one in ten people develop atrial fibrillation (AF) after an MI.

In AF, the atria beat up to 400 times per minute. So, they have time to only partly contract. The atrial and ventricular contractions are uncoordinated and the force of the contractions varies considerably. Because the heart pumps less effectively, AF causes breathlessness, palpitations and dizziness.

Initially, a person usually experiences isolated attacks of AF. Often, attacks become increasingly persistent and may eventually cause complications. For example, AF may underlie up to a quarter of strokes and triples the risk of heart failure. Ask your doctor or nurse to measure your pulse. Everyone who has an irregular pulse should have an ECG whether or not they experience symptoms.

Treating arrhythmias

Mild arrhythmias may not need treatment. Your doctor may recommend surgery or drugs (antiarrhythmics) to slow the heart if your arrhythmia causes serious symptoms or if you're at increased risk of heart failure, stroke or cardiac arrest.

During AF, the heart does not pump blood completely out of the chambers. So, blood may pool and clot. Fragments of these clots may travel from the heart and block an artery, causing a stroke or heart attack. Some people with arrhythmias receive medicines to reduce the risk of clots.

Pacemakers accelerate dangerously slow heart rate. A pacemaker is a small, battery-operated device usually implanted under the skin of your chest. When sensors detect abnormal heart rhythm, the pacemaker sends electrical pulses that restore a normal heartbeat.

In people at high risk of ventricular fibrillation, surgeons may insert an implantable cardioverter defibrillator under the skin in the chest or destroy small areas of heart tissue that generate the arrhythmia. Discuss the most appropriate treatment with your cardiologist and check out the information from the BHF and other patient groups.

Stable angina

When the heart works harder – during exercise or at times of heightened emotion, for example – narrowed coronary arteries mean that the heart's demand for oxygen can exceed supply. This imbalance causes chest pain or discomfort. Nitroglycerin (also called glyceryl trinitrate or GTN) opens the vessels supplying the heart, so alleviating the pain.

You place the GTN tablet, or spray the medicine, under your tongue to get the drug into your bloodstream rapidly. Rest also restores the balance and so alleviates the pain. However, some arteries narrowed by more than 70 per cent can trigger angina at rest.

Several other conditions can trigger angina, for example:

- nocturnal angina, where some people suffer an attack at night;
- angina decubitus, where lying down may trigger angina because gravity redistributes the body's fluids, which makes the heart work harder;

- severe hypertension;
- abnormal, narrow or leaking aortic valves;
- thickening of the walls of the heart chambers (cardiomyopathy).

Most people with angina report heaviness, tightness, pressure or pain in the centre of the chest or beneath the breastbone that generally lasts between 2 and 15 minutes. The pain, which can be severe, may spread from the chest to the left shoulder and arm to the neck or left jaw, throat, teeth, back or stomach. Some people feel nauseous or breathless, or both.

Identify your angina triggers by keeping a diary of when your symptoms emerged, how you felt and what you were doing. Triggers may include:

- exercise
- strong emotions
- large meals
- rapid changes in temperature
- sleep deprivation
- severe anaemia: ask your doctor to check, especially if you're a vegetarian or vegan (meat is the best natural source of iron) or lose a lot of blood due to heavy menstrual periods.

Keeping a diary can help you identify ways to self-manage angina, such as pacing your activities and setting goals. Your cardiac rehabilitation team or GP can help, such as advising about safe levels of physical exertion, including sex. You should also discuss ways to manage your stress, anxiety or depression and tell your GP or cardiac team as soon as the pattern of your angina changes. The angina diary will help.

Drugs for angina

Apart from alleviating the attack, you should use your anti-angina treatment before any planned exercise or exertion. Because nitrates open blood vessels, they can cause flushing, headache and light-headedness, in which case sit down or find something to hold on to.

Your doctor will probably suggest you take either a beta-blocker or a calcium channel blocker to prevent angina attacks. If the beta-blocker does not control angina adequately or you develop side effects, you can switch to the calcium channel blocker, or vice versa. Some people need both a beta-blocker and a calcium channel blocker. Your doctor may suggest other medicines or surgery if, for example, side effects remain a problem.

Other complications of an MI

Several other complications can follow in the wake of an MI:

- In pericarditis, the heart attack inflames the pericardium, the thin sac-like membrane covering the heart. The pericardium helps stop the heart from moving when you're active.
- Sometimes a heart weakened by an MI, arrhythmia or several other cardiac conditions suddenly does not pump enough blood to meet the body's needs. This can cause the symptoms of shock (Table 5 overleaf). 'Cardiogenic shock' is fatal unless treated immediately and a leading cause of death among people in hospital after an MI. Shock can arise from several causes. If you think someone is in shock, call 999 or get medical assistance immediately.

Table 5 Symptoms of shock

Confusion or lack of alertness
Loss of consciousness
Sudden and persistently rapid heartbeat
Weak pulse
Sweating
Pale skin
Rapid breathing
Reduced (or no) urine output
Cool hands and feet

- A heart attack can punch holes through the wall separating the ventricles (septal rupture). So, the ventricles can't pump efficiently. MIs can also damage the muscles anchoring the bicuspid (mitral) and tricuspid valves (Figure 2). So, blood doesn't flow correctly. Both these problems can trigger cardiogenic shock.

Depression and other psychiatric problems

Depression is common after heart attacks and unstable angina, and increases the risk of death in the next few months between four- and sevenfold. Furthermore, deaths from cardiovascular disease, lethal arrhythmias and heart attacks rise immediately after intensely stressful disasters such as earthquakes and terrorist attacks.

So, don't underestimate depression. It's more than feeling 'down in the dumps'. It's profound, debilitating mental and physical lethargy, a pervasive sense of worthlessness and intense, deep, unshakeable sadness.

You need to get help for depression, anxiety or any other psychiatric conditions, whether these emerge before or after your heart attack. People with depression may lack the motivation to take their life-saving medicines as suggested by their doctor or to make the lifestyle changes that cut the chances of further heart disease.

Don't dismiss antidepressants or drugs to alleviate anxiety out of hand. It's often difficult to plan the best way of reducing your risk of heart disease in particular or of tackling your life problems when you're carrying the burden imposed by depression or anxiety. While drugs don't cure the problem, medicines may offer you a 'window of opportunity' to improve your control of your heart disease and deal with other issues.

A counsellor can help you and your partner identify and manage the practical, psychological and emotional challenges that arise when living with chronic heart disease. Ask your GP or contact the British Association for Counselling and Psychotherapy (<www.bacp. co.uk>). Try to find a counsellor or therapist who has experience helping people with heart disease.

Returning to work

Returning to work helps reduce the risk of depression – partly because your life is getting back to normal. People usually return to work after a doctor's review at least two months after the heart attack. If tests show only minimal heart damage you may be able to return to work sooner. People who have survived a cardiac arrest or undergone CABG usually take longer off work.

Persistent symptoms – such as angina and breathlessness – and depression may reduce the chance of returning to work or at least delay your return. People who believe that stress at work caused their heart attack will probably be reluctant to return. Other people believe that they need to 'take things easy' – which means giving up their job.

Doctors and employers are more likely to 'allow' a person to go back to a sedentary job (and to return quickly) than to manual labour. However, very few jobs ban a return, although you may need a medical examination or an exercise test.

Your cardiac rehabilitation programme should include advice about returning to work. The therapist may assess the workplace or suggest 'work-hardening'. You could begin with half-days at work and light or less challenging duties, gradually building up over two to three weeks. You may need additional rest periods. Check with your doctor and the licensing authority (e.g. the DVLA or DVA) whether it's safe for you to start driving again.

Cardiac rehabilitation programmes

Most MI survivors join a cardiac rehabilitation programme, usually starting four to eight weeks after the heart attack. People who have undergone or are waiting for CABG, revascularization or other heart operations, or who suffer from heart failure or angina, may also join a cardiac rehabilitation programme. The cardiac rehabilitation team may include a cardiologist, specialist cardiac nurse, physiotherapist, exercise specialist, occupational therapist, dietician and psychologist.

Typically, the programme includes lifestyle advice, including how to manage stress, anxiety and depression and exercise. Indeed, exercise programmes for cardiac rehabilitation reduce all-cause and cardiovascular mortality by about a quarter among MI survivors. You'll set goals and be advised on when you can return to work, start to drive again and resume your sex life. They'll also help you understand the risks and benefits of treatment.

Typically, you'll go once or twice a week for about six to eight weeks. If you've not been invited to a cardiac rehabilitation programme, ask your hospital or GP. However, while the rehabilitation programme lasts a few months, changes in exercise, diet and smoking cessation should last the rest of your life.

7

Preventing another heart attack

Your chances of surviving an MI are better than ever. But, as we've seen, having one heart attack means you're much more likely to suffer another. So, to survive long term you should take your medicines as suggested by your doctor and follow a heart-healthy lifestyle. For example, INTERHEART identified four factors that reduce your risk of suffering a heart attack. These links emerged for the first MI. However, because you're at particularly high risk after a heart attack, the benefits will probably be even more marked than these figures suggest.

- Not smoking reduced the risk of suffering the first MI by 65 per cent.
- Eating fruit and vegetables daily reduced MI risk by 30 per cent.
- Moderate exercise (walking, cycling or gardening) or strenuous exercise (jogging, football and vigorous swimming) for at least four hours a week cut the risk by 14 per cent. (Always check with your doctor before starting exercise after an MI.)
- Regular alcohol consumption (three or more times a week) reduced MI risk by 9 per cent.

The healthier your lifestyle the lower the risk:

- Not smoking and eating fruit and vegetables daily reduced MI risk by 76 per cent.
- Not smoking, eating fruit and vegetables daily and regular exercise cut MI risk by 79 per cent.
- Not smoking, eating fruit and vegetables daily, regular exercise and regular alcohol consumption cut MI risk by 81 per cent.

Quit smoking

Smoking causes around half of all cases of heart disease. Unfortunately, on some measures, nicotine is more addictive than heroin or cocaine and fewer than one smoker in 30 quits each year. More than half of those who quit relapse within a year.

Withdrawal symptoms – such as irritation, restlessness, anxiety, sleeplessness and intense cravings – generally abate over about two weeks. If you cannot tough it out, nicotine replacement therapy (NRT) 'tops up' levels in the blood, without exposing you to the other harmful chemicals, and increases your chances of quitting by between 50 and 100 per cent. Patches reduce withdrawal symptoms over a relatively long time, but start alleviating symptoms slowly. Nicotine chewing gum, lozenges, inhalers and nasal sprays act more quickly, but don't last as long. Talk to your pharmacist or GP to find the right combination. Doctors can prescribe other treatments – but you still need to be motivated to quit.

Many people have quit using e-cigarettes. These don't contain most of the toxic chemicals linked to cancer or heart disease. But as these deliver nicotine, e-cigarettes remain addictive and we still don't know if there are any long-term health risks. So, e-cigarettes can take you a large step towards kicking the habit. But don't stop there.

Tips to help you quit

- Set a quit date, when you will stop completely.
- Try to quit abruptly. If you can't, cutting back seems to increase the likelihood that you will eventually quit. But don't stop when you cut back.
- Plan ahead. For a couple of weeks before you quit, note when and where you light up, then find alternatives or avoid the trigger.
- Try to find something to take your mind off smoking. If you find car journeys boring without a cigarette, try an audio book, a music CD or radio play.
- Note how much money you save and spend at least some of it on something for yourself.
- Tackle stress.
- Hypnosis can increase the chances of quitting smoking almost fivefold. Contact the British Association of Medical Hypnosis (<www.bamh.org.uk/>).

If you still cannot quit, ask your GP or practice nurse about NHS anti-smoking clinics, which offer advice, support and, when appropriate, NRT. You can obtain a free 'quit smoking' support pack from the NHS Smoking Helpline (tel. 0800 022 4332).

Nicotine is incredibly addictive and, not surprisingly, most smokers make three or four attempts to quit before they succeed. Regard any relapse as temporary, set another quit date and try again. Try to identify why you relapsed and how to prevent the problem. As the old health promotion advertisement suggests, 'Don't give up on giving up.'

Reducing blood pressure

Typically, realistic lifestyle changes reduce diastolic blood pressure by 2–3 mmHg. But some people do much better – especially when they combine several lifestyle changes (Table 6).

Nevertheless, most people need to take antihypertensives to reduce their blood pressure to safe levels. There's not space here to discuss the pros and cons of each. So, talk to your doctor and check out NHS Choices (<www.nhs.uk/>) and patient groups' websites. This diversity means, for example, if you suffer, or are at risk of, a side effect doctors can usually find an alternative.

Taking antihypertensives reduces the risk of stroke by up to two-fifths, CHD by a fifth and major cardiovascular

Table 6 Lifestyle changes' impact on blood pressure

Lifestyle change	Reduction in systolic blood pressure
Maintain BMI between 20 and 25 kg/m²	5–10 mmHg per 10 kg weight loss
Eat a diet rich in fruit, vegetables and low-fat dairy products, and low in saturated and total fat	8–14 mmHg
Reduce salt consumption to less than 2.4 g sodium (less than 6 g salt)	2–8 mmHg
Take regular aerobic activity (e.g. brisk walking for at least 30 minutes a day)	4–9 mmHg
Drink 21 units a week or less (men) or 14 units a week or less (women)	2–4 mmHg

events (stroke, MI, heart failure or death from any cardiovascular cause) by up to just over a quarter, depending on the drug and dose. However, a single antihypertensive controls blood pressure adequately in, at most, a third of patients. So, most people need at least two antihypertensives. Many people need at least three. While they can save your life, antihypertensives can cause side effects. Lifestyle modifications can, however, lower blood pressure as much as a single hypertensive.

Tackling salt

Salt drives blood pressure up. So, your cardiac team will probably tell you to reduce your salt consumption. (They will recommend an intake that's right for you.) You can tell many snacks are salty – crisps, nuts and so on. But many foods contain large amounts of hidden salt, including some soups, bread, biscuits, processed meat, cheese, stock cubes and even ice cream. So read the label and:

- avoid foods – such as smoked meat and fish – that are high in salt;
- add as little salt as you can during baking and cooking;
- banish the salt cellar from the table;
- ask restaurants and take-aways for 'no salt';
- use low-salt ketchup, pickles, mustard, yeast extract, stock cubes and so on;
- avoid foods that include a chemical name that includes sodium, such as disodium phosphate, monosodium glutamate or sodium nitrate;
- choose meals and sandwiches with less than 1.25 g of salt per meal;
- choose individual foods with less than 0.75 grams of salt per serving.

Fat

Atherosclerotic plaques (page 8) are rich in cholesterol. However, the amount of cholesterol in your blood depends more on the amount of saturated (animal) fat in your diet than the amount of cholesterol-rich foods you eat. The liver converts saturated fat into cholesterol. So, eat less food high in saturated fat. Foods with more than 5 g of saturated fat per 100 g are high in fat. If changing to a low-fat diet isn't sufficient, you may need to take medicines. However, these are an addition to a low-fat diet rather than a replacement.

Numerous foods – including cheese, cream, beef, lamb and mutton – contain trans fats (fatty acids), which gram for gram increase heart disease risk more than saturated fats. Heating vegetable oil to fry foods and some food processing methods also create trans fatty acids. These artificial trans fats seem to be much more harmful to the heart than 'natural' trans fats. Biscuits, pies, cakes and some margarines and other spreads often contain hydrogenated (also called trans-unsaturated) fats. So, look for 'low in trans' or 'virtually trans free' foods and check the ingredients. Foods containing hydrogenated fats or hydrogenated vegetable oils almost always contain trans fats.

Fibre and whole grains

Dietary fibre (roughage) is the part of plants that humans can't digest. There are two types:

- Insoluble fibre remains largely intact as it moves through your digestive system, but eases defecation.
- Soluble fibre dissolves in water in the gut, forming a gel that soaks up fats.

Regularly eating foods rich in soluble fibre – including oats and oat bran, fruit and vegetables, nuts, beans and pulses such as peas, soya, lentils and chickpeas – helps reduce the amount of saturated fat you absorb from your diet.

Whole grains – such as wheat, rye, barley, oats and rice – are an especially good source of fibre. An outer layer that is rich in fibre (bran) covers the nutrient-packed 'germ'. Food manufacturers refine grain by removing the bran and germ, and keep the white central area (endosperm). So, whole grain contains up to 75 per cent more nutrients than refined cereals.

Regularly eating whole grains as part of a low-fat diet and a healthy lifestyle cuts the risk of heart disease and type 2 diabetes by almost a third. Whole grains release sugar slowly into your blood. This, along with the high fibre content, means that you feel fuller for longer. So, you're less likely to snack. Eat more foods with 'whole' in front of the grain's name – such as wholewheat pasta and whole oats.

A very British alcohol unit

In the UK, a 'unit' contains 8 g (or 10 ml) of alcohol. A standard bottle (750 ml) of 12 per cent wine contains nine units – so there are three units in a large (250 ml) glass of wine. A pint of 5 per cent beer or cider also contains three units. So, that's 24 g of alcohol. A US 'drink' contains 14 g of alcohol – just under two British units.

Alcohol and heart attacks

Drinking small amounts of alcohol cuts the risk of heart disease. A review of 84 studies found that compared to abstaining, drinking 2.5–14.9 g (in other words, less than two units) of alcohol a day reduced the risk of:

- CHD by about a quarter;
- death from cardiovascular disease by about a quarter;
- death from CHD by about a fifth;
- stroke by about a fifth;
- death from stroke by about a seventh.

However, 15 g of alcohol a day is less than a pint of beer. Drinking more than this soon becomes hazardous. For example, binge drinking (consuming more than 50 g on at least one day a week – that's more than about six units or two pints of strong beer) almost doubles the risk of heart attack and coronary death. Furthermore, heavy drinking over a long time (usually 5–15 years) can directly damage the heart, leading to heart failure.

If you're worried about your drinking call the national drink helpline on 0800 917 8282. Ask your GP or cardiac team about how much you can safely drink.

Exercise

A sudden bout of unaccustomed exercise can trigger heart attacks. In one study, short-term bouts of exercise increased the risk of suffering a heart attack by 3.5 times and sudden cardiac death by about five times. Even sexual activity almost trebled heart attack risk.

On the other hand, each work-out over a week roughly halved the risk of heart attack associated with short-term exercise and sexual activity, and reduced the risk of sudden cardiac death by about a third. So, discuss the amount of physical activity you need with your doctor.

Immediately after a heart attack, your cardiologist, nurse or physiotherapist will suggest beginning with gentle activity and gradually increasing the intensity. This advice is tailored to each person. In general, the BHF suggests taking things easy for the first two or three days after your discharge following a heart attack. You should do about the same amount of moving around and exercise indoors as during your last few days in hospital. Make sure that you get enough rest.

Provided your doctor doesn't tell you otherwise, you can then perform light tasks around the home, such as making drinks and light snacks, going up and down stairs a few times a day, and gentle walking. Most heart attack survivors can start doing light housework – such as washing up and dusting – when they feel able. After a few weeks, you can probably use a vacuum cleaner, carry the laundry and do light gardening. But avoid digging and heavy lifting. If you're in any doubt or you feel unwell at any time, immediately contact your doctor.

Gradually increase your physical activity over the next few weeks. But don't push yourself. Many people tire easily after a heart attack. The tiredness usually declines as your strength and confidence return. If you suffer angina or feel breathless you must stop and rest. Always carry your anti-angina treatments with you and use them as suggested by your doctor.

Walking – ideally on flat ground – is a good exercise during the first few weeks after a heart attack. (Check with the cardiologist or cardiac rehabilitation team what's right for you.) However, exercising after a large

meal, when it is very cold or very hot or at high altitudes can place additional strain on your heart.

After a few weeks, and provided the medical team
agrees, you can probably return to using a treadmill,
jogging or swimming (if you swam regularly before
your heart attack). However, the pool should be reason-
ably warm. If you experience pain in your chest, arm,
jaw or shoulder or you are unusually breathless, you
should stop exercising and see your doctor.

Lose weight

Abdominal obesity (page 16) increases the risk of suffering a heart attack. So, your waist size can tell you
whether your health is at risk (Table 7).

Losing weight is not easy – whatever the latest fad
diets would have you believe. However, the following
tips may help:

- Agree realistic targets with your team, such as losing
  0.5 kg (1 lb) a week until you reach your target BMI.

Table 7 Waist sizes linked to health risk

	Waist size putting health at risk	*Waist size putting health at high risk*
Men	Over 94 cm (37 inches)	Over 102 cm (40 inches)
Women	Over 80 cm (32 inches)	Over 88 cm (35 inches)
South Asian men		Over 90 cm (36 inches)
South Asian women		Over 80 cm (32 inches)

Source: British Heart Foundation.

- Exercise and a healthy diet will help you lose weight. So, try to stick to them.
- Keep a food diary and record everything you eat and drink for a couple of weeks. The odd biscuit here, extra glass of wine or full-fat latte adds up. A food diary can also help you see if you're eating fatty or high-salt food without realizing.
- Don't let a slip-up derail your diet. Identify why you indulged – what were the triggers? A particular occasion? Do you comfort eat? Develop strategies to stop the problem.

If all this fails, try talking to your GP or pharmacist. A growing number of medicines may help kick-start your weight loss. You'll still need to change your life-style. However, they help put you on the right course towards weight loss.

Vaccination

Influenza isn't a bad cold. Flu is potentially fatal, especially for older people and those with certain serious medical conditions, including heart disease. Ask your GP if you and your close family should have the jab.

Complementary and alternative medicine

Few areas of medicine attract as much controversy as complementary and alternative medicines (CAMs). They're popular: in one study, one in ten people with CHD used CAMs for their cardiac problems or other illnesses. Many people find CAMs relaxing. We've seen that emotions and stress can trigger angina. Relaxation therapies – including progressive muscle relaxation, meditation, yoga, assertiveness training and anger control techniques – reduce blood pressure.

Some herbs undoubtedly help the heart. The white foxglove yields a drug called digoxin that doctors still prescribe for some cases of heart failure and atrial fibrillation. Nevertheless, many doctors and nurses remain cynical. Certainly few CAMs undergo the same rigorous scrutiny as modern medicines. But clinical studies are expensive and pharmaceutical companies fund most trials. No evidence of effectiveness isn't necessarily the same as evidence of no effect.

Cynics add that the placebo effect accounts for most of CAMs' benefits. In other words, if you think that treatment will work and you relax, you'll probably feel better. However, the placebo effect also contributes to the benefits of conventional medicines.

A common misconception

There's a common misconception that because CAMs are natural they are safe. But always check that it's safe to take a supplement or herbal treatment; some can, for example, interact with other drugs or might be potentially hazardous if you have certain medical conditions:

- Asian ginseng may be unsuitable for diabetics.
- St John's wort (used for depression) can interact with the contraceptive pill and with warfarin.
- Garlic makes the blood less likely to clot.
- High doses of vitamin E can interact with anticoagulant or antiplatelet medications, such as aspirin and warfarin, and increase the risk of bleeding.
- Vitamin E combined with other antioxidants – such as vitamin C, selenium and beta-carotene – can under-

mine the effectiveness of some drugs that tackle harmful fat levels in your blood.

Not all products include the detailed information you need to take the supplement safely. So talk to your doctor or cardiac nurse before trying a CAM. Indeed, rather than treating yourself using herbs, it's usually better to consult a qualified practitioner. Contact the National Institute of Medical Herbalists (<www.nimh.org.uk>).

8

Heart attacks and the family

After a heart attack, family members may treat the survivor with kid gloves. But to recover fully, a person who has had a heart attack needs to get back in the swing of everyday life. Walking the tightrope between not letting you do anything and allowing you to do too much, dealing with the practical problems, as well as the sobering thought you might have died and your fears for the future, can make the weeks after your heart attack especially difficult.

Meanwhile, your partner and family may fear being left alone if you die, they may worry that sex could trigger an attack and may feel guilty about taking any personal time out. This can, obviously, place a considerable strain on your relationship – just when you need your partner the most.

So you, your partner and, when appropriate, other family members should discuss what you should do, and when, with the cardiac rehabilitation team, the GP and the district or cardiac nurses. In some parts of the country, you and your partner may receive a visit from a cardiac liaison or BHF nurse, who can answer your questions and offer advice.

Several studies suggest that a strong, supportive marriage and other 'satisfying' social relationships improve cardiovascular health, reduce premature death from heart disease and improve your chances of surviving an MI. A close family and strong marriage can give patients an especially powerful 'reason to live'. Obviously, people benefit from social, practical and emotional support. Indeed, the benefits of marriage persist for many years, which probably reflects the impact of lifestyle changes.

Your partner can help by, for instance, changing the shopping list or exercising together. He or she can ignore bad moods triggered by nicotine withdrawal, boost your motivation and watch for harmful behaviours, such as offering a gentle reminder if you start eating unhealthy food regularly or forget to take your medicine.

Nevertheless, partners need to tread a fine line. A spouse's support can reinforce his or her partner's efforts to tackle unhealthy behaviours. Control – trying to persuade a partner to adopt healthy behaviours when he or she is unwilling or unable – reduces the likelihood that the survivor will make the changes and undermines mental health.

Remembering medication

Some people may not take their medicines because they feel the drugs are unnecessary, because they deny that they're ill or because depression has sapped their motivation. Other people don't fully appreciate the risks that they're running by not taking their medication. A full and frank discussion of your concerns, and the risks and benefits, should help you understand why you need to take the medicines that could, quite literally, save your life. If you feel that you're developing side effects, speak to your GP: there are many drugs for heart disease and there is usually an alternative.

Often, however, it's by accident that people don't follow their doctor's advice. They may misunderstand instructions, become confused or simply forget. In these cases, adherence aids (such as a box that allows you to organize your tablets day by day) could help, as could simplifying your treatment. (Ask your doctor to check that you really need all the drugs.) People with physical disabilities may experience difficulties opening packaging or swallowing medication. Pharmacists may be able to suggest alternative packaging or dosing forms, such as avoiding 'child-resistant' pill bottles or using liquid formulations.

Establish a routine for taking your medicines. Some partners and family members write a list of the medicines the patient takes and when. You can tick the list when you've taken them. This also helps you to remember the medicines you're taking when you need treatment for heart disease or another condition. Some medicines can interact with another drug, either causing side effects or undermining the effectiveness of one or both drugs. You could give this list to an unfamiliar doctor (for example, if you're on holiday), to A&E staff and to pharmacists if you're buying drugs without a prescription.

Holiday

A few days away helps you and your family relax. But plan your holiday carefully:

- Avoid places that are very hot or very cold.
- Avoid high altitudes. There's less oxygen in the air at high altitudes. So, your heart has to work harder.
- Check that the accommodation isn't on too steep a hill or slope, or too far from restaurants, shops and

entertainment. (Google Maps with Street View may help.)

- Levels of pollution, which can exacerbate heart problems and even trigger MIs, are much higher in some other parts of the world than in the UK: it might be worth checking the air quality of any city you plan to visit.

- Try to avoid stress. Try going to a destination that you've visited recently to reduce the risk of unwelcome surprises and make sure you leave plenty of time to reach the airport or destination.

- Don't carry heavy bags or rush around. People with angina or some other problems may be able to get transport around the terminal.

- Always check with your cardiologist, GP or rehabilitation nurse (as well as the airline and travel insurance company) that it is safe to fly.

- If you have a pacemaker, you can bypass security systems in shops and airports that could, in rare cases, affect the device. You should have a pacemaker registration card that you always carry with you that allows you to bypass the systems.

- Check that your travel insurance offers adequate coverage. Have information about local emergency and other health services in your destination – ask your tour operator. In the UK, you can check using NHS Choices.

- Take sufficient medicines – remember, a repeat prescription won't be available at the end of a phone. Have a supply in your hand luggage and in your suitcase, and take a list of all your drugs and doses. Check for any restrictions about bringing medicines (bought from a pharmacy or on prescription) into your destination. Some painkillers can pose a particular problem in certain countries, for example. Check with the relevant consulate or embassy before you leave home.

Sex and the heart attack survivor

Most people return to their 'normal' sex life after a heart attack. However, sex can, like any physical activity, increase heart rate and blood pressure, which may cause breathlessness and chest pain. If you make an uncomplicated recovery, you can usually start having sex again about four weeks after the heart attack, provided you feel comfortable. If you're in any doubt, check with your cardiologist, GP or rehabilitation nurse. The BHF provides DVDs and booklets about heart disease and sex life.

If physical activity tends to trigger angina, don't have sex after a heavy meal, keep the bedroom warm and avoid cold sheets. Don't drink too much alcohol, create a relaxing atmosphere and get into a comfortable position. You may find that it helps if your partner takes a more active role. Keep your anti-angina treatment by the bed.

Stress following a heart attack can cause impotence. So a romantic mood and tackling any psychological issues can help reinvigorate a sex life that stalls after a heart attack. Talking to a counsellor may help.

Some drugs or diseases can affect your sex drive or cause impotence. Speak to your GP if you think a medicine or a poorly controlled ailment could be causing impotence. Switching treatment may resolve the problem. You may be able to take a drug for impotence. So, speak to your doctor and never buy any medicine over the internet.

A word to carers

Caring for a heart attack survivor can be physically demanding and emotionally draining. So, to help look after your partner you need to look after yourself.

Try to rest while your partner is resting and to get a good night's sleep yourself. You should follow the advice offered by the cardiologist, GP or rehabilitation nurse about your partner's activity. Don't offer to do more than this. Your good intentions could hinder his or her recovery and place an unnecessary burden on your shoulders. In the first few days after the MI, try to limit the number of visitors you have and how long they stay for. Make sure you have time to yourself.

A heart attack can leave your partner mentally and emotionally devastated. He or she may live over-shadowed by the fear of another heart attack, may be afraid of dying, or may worry about not being able to take part in activities that he or she previously enjoyed. Not surprisingly, heart attack survivors may feel depressed, angry, guilty and bad-tempered, which can place a strain on relationships. (If you think your partner's daily life is being affected by depression or anxiety, gently try to get him or her to see the GP.) Partners of people who suffer a heart attack often also harbour feelings of anger, guilt and resentment. Don't bottle these feelings up. Talk to the patient, friends and family or a counsellor.

You could join a local or on-line patient group. Groups run by the British Cardiac Patients Association (<www.bcpa.co.uk>) provide advice, information and support to help anyone who has had a heart condition. The BHF hosts an online community (<http://community.bhf.org.uk>), while Carers Direct is a national information, advice and support service for carers in England (<www.nhs.uk/carersdirect>; tel. 0808 802 0202).

A final word

Doctors, scientists and public health officials have made impressive progress tackling heart disease over the last few years. Fewer people than a generation ago now suffer a heart attack and the chances of surviving are better than ever. Nevertheless, you can't rely on drugs and surgery to pick up the pieces after an MI. You need to take steps to reduce your risk of suffering another heart attack and live as full and rich a life as possible after your MI, by making lifestyle changes and following your doctor's advice. An MI doesn't need to break your – or your family's – heart.